# CILANTRO AND

# CORIANDER

MARIAN KIM

# CONTENTS

# 1

# PROPERTIES

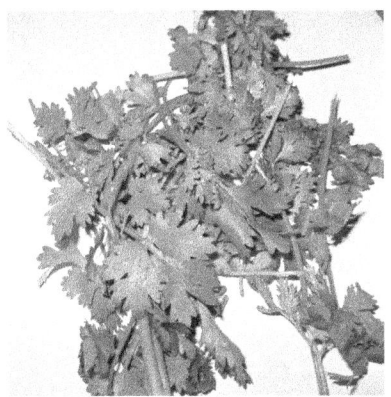

Cilantro is the name used to refer to the leaves while coriander refers to the seeds of this plant.

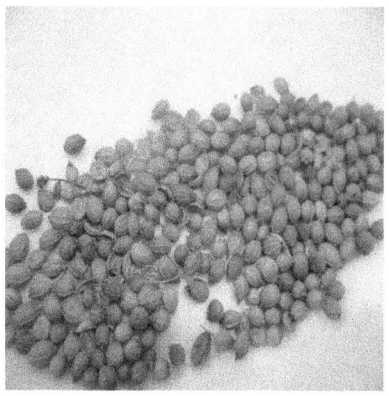

**Scientific name:** Corandrum sativum

**Other names:** Chinese parsley, dhania

**Nutrients:** Dietary fiber and vitamins A, C and K. It also contains minerals like iron, calcium, copper, magnesium, manganese, sodium and potassium. It also contains flavonoids and other phytonutrients.

## Properties

Anti-inflammatory properties

Anti-cancer properties

Antimicrobial (antibacterial, antifungal) properties

Analgesic (pain relieving) effects

*, *, *, *, *

# 2

# USES

## Uses of Cilantro

The uses of cilantro include:

**Reduce high cholesterol**

Cilantro is used to reduce high cholesterol levels.

**Arthritis treatment**

Cilantro is used to treat arthritis since it has an analgesic effect.

**Varicose vein treatment**

Cilantro is used to treat varicose veins since it has a high content of bioflavonoids.

**Hemorrhoid treatment**

Cilantro is used to treat hemorrhoids since it has a high content of bioflavonoids.

## Conjunctivitis treatment

Cilantro is beneficial for conjunctivitis since it reduces the irritation.

## Aphrodisiac

Cilantro can be used as an aphrodisiac.

# Uses of Coriander

The uses of coriander include:

## Urinary tract infection treatment

Coriander is useful for treating urinary tract infections (UTIs) since it has antibacterial properties. It is also used to prevent UTIs.

## Minor skin infection treatment

Coriander is used to treat minor skin infections caused by bacteria and fungi due to its antibacterial and antifungal properties.

## Digestive aid

Coriander aids digestion. Coriander tea is also used to treat indigestion.

## Flatulence treatment

Coriander reduces flatulence.

## Managing irritable bowel syndrome (IBS)

Coriander tea has helped persons with irritable bowel syndrome by calming intestinal spasms.

## Reduce high blood sugar

Coriander is used to reduce high blood sugar levels.

## Reduce high blood pressure

Coriander can also be used to lower blood pressure.

## Muscle pain relief

Coriander is used to relieve muscle pains. It also has muscle relaxant effects.

## Headache treatment

Coriander is used to treat headaches.

## Stiffness

Coriander is used to relieve stiffness.

## Nausea prevention

Coriander juice is used to prevent nausea. It is also used for morning sickness.

## Alzheimer's disease prevention

Coriander can be used to prevent Alzheimer's disease and memory loss since it prevents the accumulation of heavy metals in the body.

## Diarrhea and dysentery treatment

Dry coriander is used to treat diarrhea. Coriander juice is used to treat dysentery.

## Colitis treatment

Coriander juice is used to treat colitis and indigestion.

## Acne prevention

Coriander juice is used to prevent the blackheads and pimples of acne when it is mixed with turmeric.

## Anxiety treatment

Some studies have shown that coriander can be used to treat anxiety due to its anxiolytic effects.

## Panic attacks treatment

Some studies have shown that coriander can be used to treat panic attacks due to its anxiolytic and sedative effects.

## Depression treatment

Some studies have shown that coriander can be used to treat depression since it can cause a mild euphoria.

### Anorexia treatment

Coriander infusion is used for anorexia since it can increase the appetite.

### Heavy periods management

Boiled coriander seeds are useful for women with heavy menstrual blood flow and hormonal mood swings.

### Breast milk induction

Coriander is used to increase the flow of milk by breastfeeding women.

### Dry skin management

Coriander can be used to manage dry skin.

### Eczema management

Coriander can be used to manage eczema.

### Halitosis management

Coriander is used to freshen the breath.

### Mouth ulcers treatment

Coriander is used to treat ulcers in the mouth.

### Antihelminthic

Coriander is used to treat worms.

### Antipyretic

Coriander is used to lower fever. It is usually mixed with milk and honey when used as antipyretic.

MARIAN KIM

*, *, *, *, *

# 3

# SAFETY PRECAUTIONS

1. Coriander can cause increased sensitivity to sunlight which can lead to sunburns and skin cancer. Persons using it should therefore apply sunscreen and wear protective clothing when in the sun.

2. Persons who are allergic to mugwort, aniseed, caraway, fennel and dill can develop allergic reactions after using coriander.

3. Persons using medications for diabetes should use cautiously or avoid coriander since it can also lower blood sugar levels.

4. Persons with low blood pressure or those using medications for high blood pressure should use cautiously or avoid coriander since it can also lower the blood pressure.

# 4

# DRUG INTERACTIONS

None noted todate.

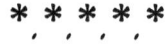

# 5

# COOKING TIPS

**Cilantro Flavor:**

Earthy piney, lemony, parsley-like or soapy to some people

**Cilantro Goes well with:**

Seafood e.g. prawns, mussels, scallops, poultry e.g. chicken, vegetables e.g. carrots, meat dishes e.g. beef, fish, fruits e.g. avocado, sauces e.g. soy sauce, salsas, salads, chutneys, chili, couscous, rice, beans, Asian, Mexican, Indian cuisine

**Cilantro Can be substituted with::**

Parsley

**Cilantro Tips:**

Fresh cilantro is best added at end of the cooking process since heat reduces its flavor and destroys its lovely green color.

MARIAN KIM

\* \* \* \* \*
, , , ,

# 6

# HERBAL RECIPES

## Coriander Tea

### Equipment

Kettle

Tea cup

***

### Ingredients

1 teaspoon of finely crushed coriander

1 cup of boiling water

Honey to taste (optional)

\*\*\*

## Instructions

1. Put the coriander in a tea cup, add the boiling water and let it steep while covered for 10 -15 minutes.

2. Add honey (if using) to suit your taste before drinking.

\*\*\*

## Tips

1. Adding ginger to this tea can help relieve abdominal pain caused by indigestion.

\*\*\*\*\*

# Coriander Juice

## Equipment

Glass bowl

\*\*\*

## Ingredients

1 tablespoon coriander

1 cup of water

\*\*\*

## Instructions

1. Soak the coriander seeds in the water overnight.

2. Strain the seeds and the coriander juice is ready for consumption.

\*\*\*

## Tips

1. Add buttermilk to the coriander juice and drink it in the morning to relieve diarrhea.

2. Add turmeric to the coriander juice and apply it to acne pimples to help clear them.

\*\*\*\*\*

# Coriander Infusion

## Equipment
Glass jar with tight fitting lid

\*\*\*

## Ingredients
1 tablespoon dried coriander

1 cup boiling water

\*\*\*

## Instructions
1. Place the herb in the glass jar and add the boiling water to fill the jar.

2. Close the lid and let the mixture steep for 4 hours to 14 hours (overnight).

3. Strain the herb and the infusion is ready for consumption.

\*\*\*

## Tips
1. Store the infusion in the refrigerator to lengthen its life.

\*\*\*\*\*

# Coriander Syrup

## Equipment

Saucepan

Jar with airtight lid

\*\*\*

## Ingredients

1 quart (1000 ml) filtered water

1 cup coriander

1 cup honey

\*\*\*

## Instructions

1. Place the water and coriander in a saucepan and bring to a boil.

2. Reduce the heat and let it simmer while it is partially covered until the volume is reduced to half the original volume.

3. Strain the mixture through a sieve or cheesecloth to remove the herbs.

4. Measure 1 pint (500 mls) of the liquid and add the honey.

5. Cook for a few minutes as you stir it so that it thickens.

6. Store the syrup in an airtight container in the fridge for up to 2 months.

\*\*\*\*\*

# Coriander Infused Oil

## Equipment

Double boiler

Large glass bowl

Sieve and cheesecloth

Sterilized dark jars

**\*\*\***

## Ingredients

16 fl oz. (500 ml) vegetable like sweet almond oil or sunflower oil

8 oz. (250 grams) coriander

**\*\*\***

## Instructions

1. Place the coriander and oil in the glass bowl ensuring that the oil covers the herbs. Simmer them in a double boiler for one hour at a temperature of around 120 degrees Fahrenheit (49 degrees Celsius). Do not let the mixture boil. You can repeat this step several times after letting the oils cool to create more concentrated herb infused oils.

2. Strain the mixture through the sieve and cheesecloth into a clean, dark jar ensuring you squeeze out as much oil as you can from the cheesecloth.

3. Label your jars and store your herb infused oils in a cool dark place or in the refrigerator and use them within 3 months.

**\*\*\*\*\***

# Cilantro Butter

## Equipment

Large glass bowl

Electric mixer or stick blender or wire whisk

Molds such as ice cube trays (optional)

**\*\*\***

## Ingredients

½ cup butter

2 tablespoons of finely minced, fresh cilantro

**\*\*\***

## Instructions

1. Place the butter in a warm place so that it can soften.

2. Put butter and cilantro in a large glass bowl and blend well until thoroughly mixed.

3. Refrigerate until it hardens. You can refrigerate it in molds or ice cube trays to give it a special shape.

**\*\*\*\*\***

# Cilantro Juice

## Equipment

Blender

\*\*\*

## Ingredients

1 cup cilantro

1 cup cucumber slices

1 inch slice of fresh ginger or ½ teaspoon ginger powder

1 cup of water

\*\*\*

## Instructions

1. Place all the ingredients in the blender and mix until you get a smooth consistency

### ###

# ABOUT THE AUTHOR

Marian Kim is an experienced alternative medicine practitioner.

# OTHER BOOKS BY THE AUTHOR

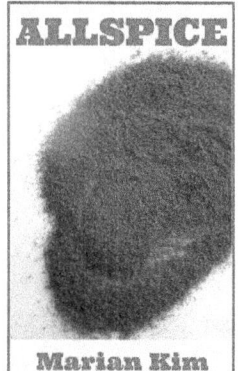

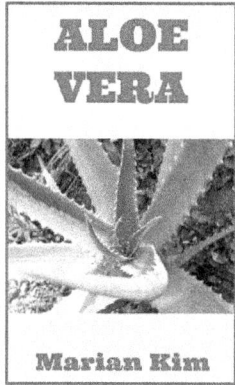

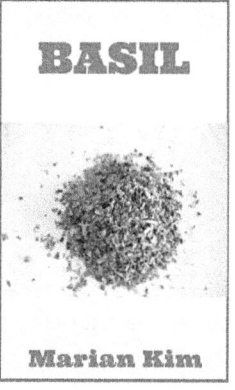

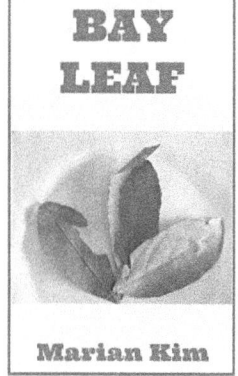

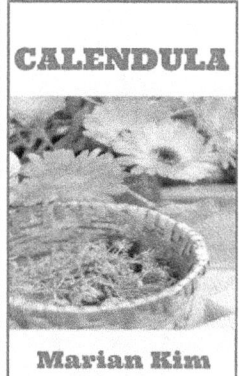

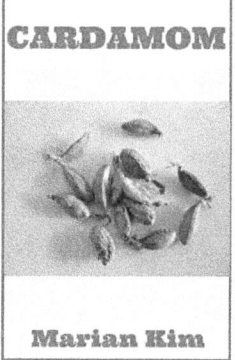

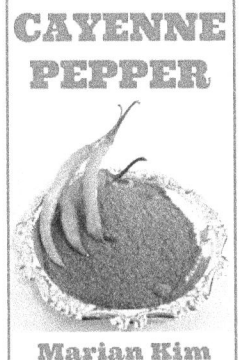

CAYENNE PEPPER

Marian Kim

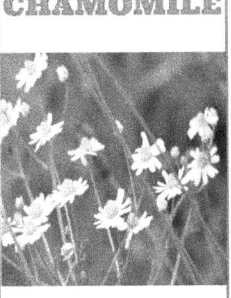

CHAMOMILE

Marian Kim

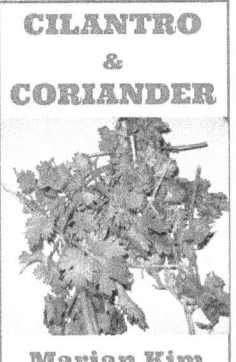

CILANTRO & CORIANDER

Marian Kim

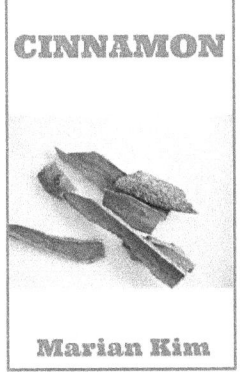

CINNAMON

Marian Kim

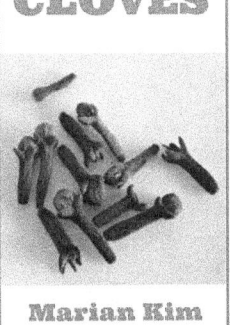

CLOVES

Marian Kim

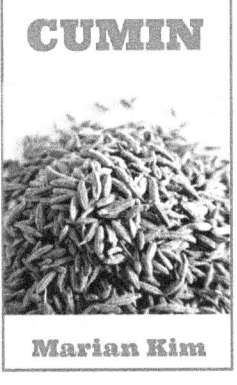

CUMIN

Marian Kim

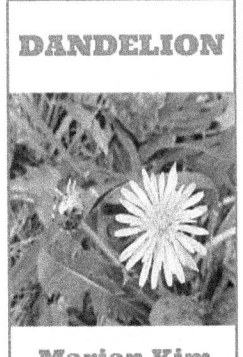

DANDELION

Marian Kim

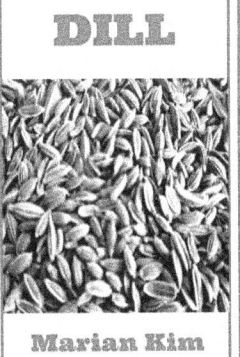

DILL

Marian Kim

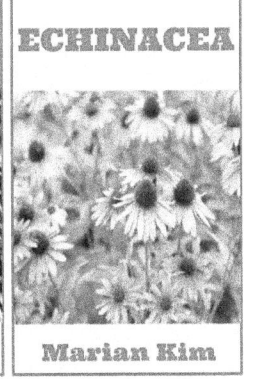

ECHINACEA

Marian Kim

**FENNEL**

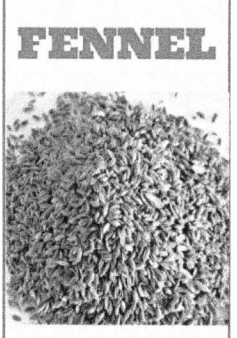

Marian Kim

**FENUGREEK**

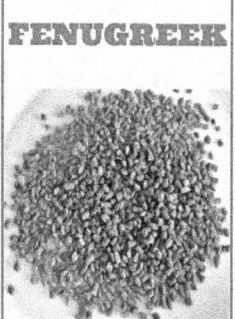

Marian Kim

**GARLIC**

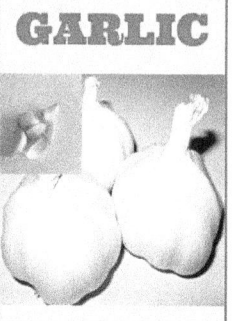

Marian Kim

**GINGER**

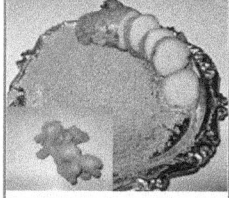

Marian Kim

**GINKGO BILOBA**

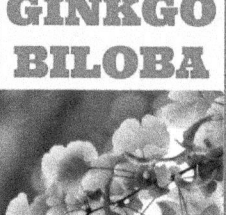

Marian Kim

**GINSENG**

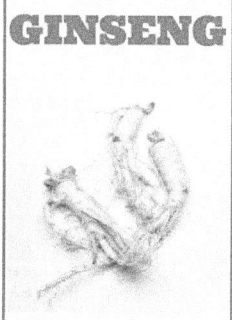

Marian Kim

**LAVENDER**

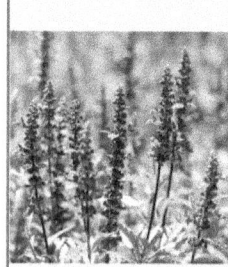

Marian Kim

**MUSTARD**

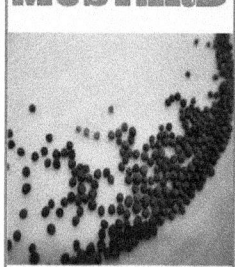

Marian Kim

**NEEM**

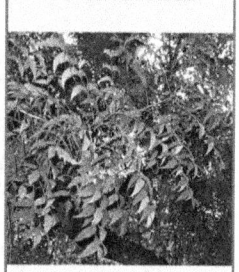

Marian Kim

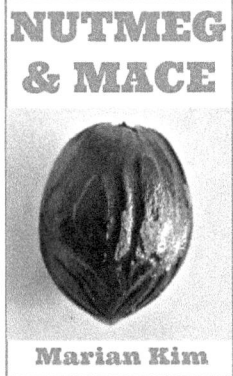

NUTMEG & MACE

Marian Kim

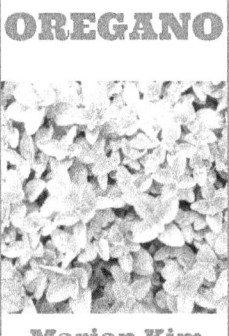

OREGANO

Marian Kim

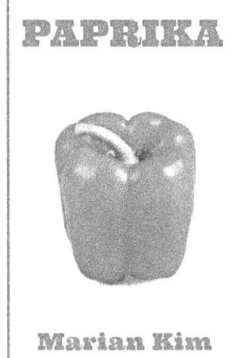

PAPRIKA

Marian Kim

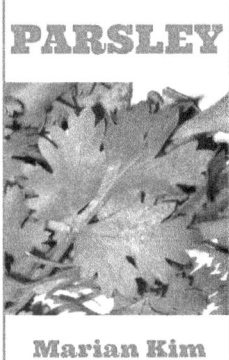

PARSLEY

Marian Kim

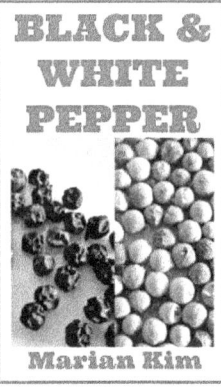

BLACK & WHITE PEPPER

Marian Kim

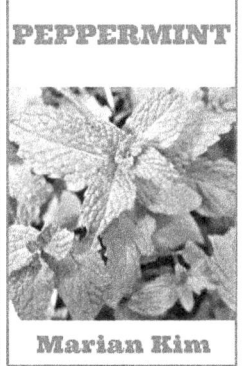

PEPPERMINT

Marian Kim

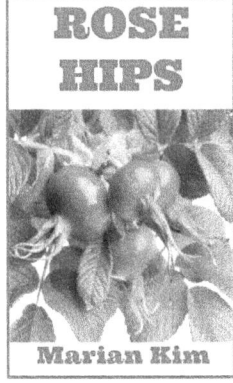

ROSE HIPS

Marian Kim

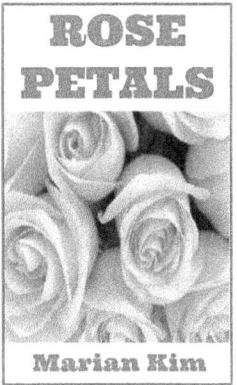

ROSE PETALS

Marian Kim

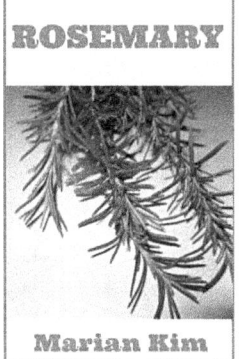

ROSEMARY

Marian Kim

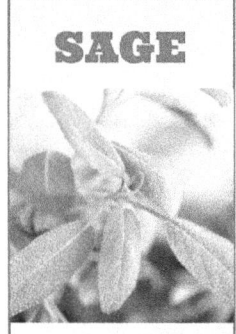

SAGE

Marian Kim

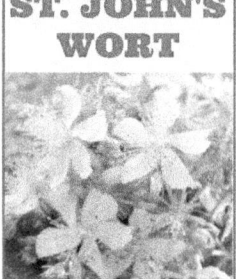

ST. JOHN'S WORT

Marian Kim

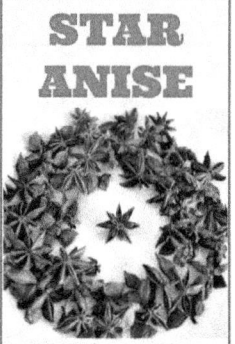

STAR ANISE

Marian Kim

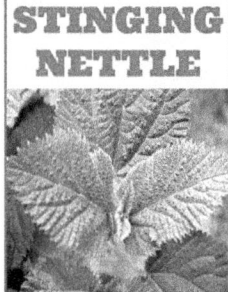

STINGING NETTLE

Marian Kim

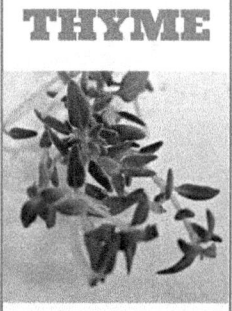

THYME

Marian Kim

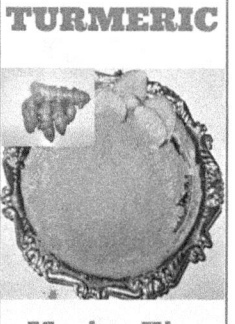

TURMERIC

Marian Kim

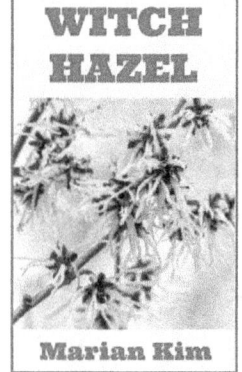

WITCH HAZEL

Marian Kim

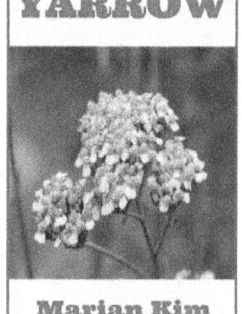

YARROW

Marian Kim

\*\*\*\*\*